Gastric Bypass Cookbook

77 Healthy and Delicious Bariatric Recipes with an Easy Guide to Being on a Weight Loss Surgery Diet

Table of Contents

Introduction

Hi! I would like to begin this book by saying that just by making it to this page shows that you have the necessary passion and deep urge to make some positive changes in your life and health. I congratulate you on that great desire inside of you that may seem insignificant at the moment, but simply "opening the door" to change, and accepting the possibilities, is always the hardest part. So once again, congratulations to you for taking this initial step! Give yourself a pat on the back, you deserve it!

According to the World Health Organization (WHO), health is a state of "complete physical, mental, and social well-being".

Health, well-being, and beauty are the most precious gifts you can give to yourself. We all have a tendency to stay fit and healthy and it's a rare gift especially in modern times where life is packed with stress and different chemicals that destroy our health in so many different ways. In such times, our number one priority in life is to stay healthy and keep our weight in check.

This book will guide you through the entire gastric bypass surgery process. In the first chapter, I will explain everything you need to know about the procedure itself. Later on, I will lead you through four different stages of the recovery process and make things much easier. And when you completely recover from the operation, you will learn how to adopt some healthy eating habits for the rest of your life. This part is particularly important because it's tough to achieve and maintain the weight you want. As someone who went through a gastric bypass surgery, you surely know this. I have found that the hardest part can be creating the right diet plan that will give you a proper nutrition and help with the weight loss process. It can be difficult physically and mentally, and it can take weeks, even months for the first results to come. For this reason, setting up your short-term and long-term goals is extremely important. We will go there together.

This book is not just a simple guide through the procedure itself. This book contains all the information you need to know in order to lose the weight and keep your results permanently in the easiest way there possibly is. This book is your guide to a full recovery after the gastric bypass surgery.

But it doesn't stop there. It was my deepest desire to give you a wide range of delicious recipes you can easily prepare without jeopardizing your health. These recipes are based on healthy foods that are allowed on each stage of your journey. Furthermore, a collection of 77 delicious recipes will satisfy your taste and food cravings.

I hope this book will make you realize that having your health and life back is nothing to be afraid of. Follow my advice and let's begin this journey together...

Luke Newman

What is a Gastric Bypass Surgery

Gastric bypass surgery is a medical procedure that will shrink your stomach and help you lose weight. This life saving procedure will permanently change the way you eat, and most importantly, change the way your digestive tract handles food. This means you that after the surgery your body will start to change and you will feel much better. But, I have to point out that in order to be 100% successful, the surgery itself will not be enough. You will have the change the way you eat and adopt some long-term diet habits. Only this will permanently help you control your body weight and make you look exactly the way you want to look. But we'll get to that later. Now, let's get back to the procedure itself.

Depending on their state, most people decide or have to go through a gastric bypass surgery. Sometimes, it's the only solution, especially if you weren't able to lose any weight through diet and exercise. However, you have to understand that a gastric bypass is not some quick fix solution for your weight problems. This is a serious medical procedure that will completely change your entire life.

After the surgery, you will have to follow a strict diet plan in order to recover from the operation. In the first couple of weeks, up to two month, your diet will be carefully planned by your nutritionist or even a doctor. It will be based mostly on liquid and soft, easy-chewable foods. These couple of weeks might be difficult especially after you're used having large portions and amounts of foods. But, trust me, it's worth it!

When your body finally recovers from the surgery, you will simply have to change your entire eating habits and diet plan. You must eat healthy foods in smaller portions, and include some moderate physical activity into your daily schedule. These rules are very important to follow. In the contrary, you will not be seeing the results you're after and you may even get some post-operation complications.

Before the surgery, your doctor will calculate your **BMI** (body mass index) and exam your overall health condition in order to determine if you're going to benefit from the surgery. A **BMI** over 40 is defined as obesity and most likely you will have to take the surgery in order to lose some weight as soon as possible due to high risk of type 2 diabetes, heart disease, and other obesity-related diseases.

After your doctor determines you will greatly benefit from this surgery, you will go through a complete physical exam that includes blood tests, gallbladder ultrasound, and other tests to determine some other medical conditions like high blood pressure or diabetes are under control. Furthermore, you will most likely be scheduled for a complete nutritional counseling or even classes where you can learn what will happen during and after the surgery. You need to learn and accept all the risks this procedure brings and make sure you're completely emotionally ready for this. Also, you will have to accept some major changes in your diet and lifestyle after the surgery.

Another important thing you will be told before the surgery is to stop smoking at least for a couple of weeks before the scheduled date. Naturally, you will have to quit smoking after the surgery as well. This unnatural habit makes a serious damage and slows down the entire recovery process.

Only after a complete and positive physical exam, you will be scheduled for the surgery. Before you blindly accept the procedure, make sure you understand everything it brings. Also, make sure to tell your doctor what types of medicines you're taking because you might be asked to stop taking them before the surgery. This information can be lifesaving, so make sure not to lie to your doctor. Follow their advice strictly without any modifications. You have to understand one thing – this is a serious operation and you have to be completely disciplined to reduce the risks it might bring.

Just like any other surgery, you will be given a complete, general anesthesia before the procedure. Naturally, the procedure will be completely painless. Now that you have fallen asleep, your surgeon will use staples and divide your stomach into two sections – smaller upper section and larger bottom section. From now on, the smaller upper section will serve as your stomach. This is where the food will go in the future. The volume of this stomach part will be around 1oz and that is the main reason you will lose weight.

After your stomach has been divided into two sections, your surgeon will make a bypass that will connect the smaller upper section and your intestines. This way, the food will go directly from your shrank stomach into your intestines resulting in less calorie absorption.

The procedure itself takes about 2-4 hours, depending on each individual, while the recovery procedure takes up to 8 weeks.

Pre-Operation Diet

Before the gastric bypass operation, you will be told to follow a strict diet plan. The reason for this is to reduce the amount of fats around liver and spleen and make the procedure less risky and easier. If, however, you don't follow the prescribed diet, your surgery will be rescheduled or even canceled. The rules of this liquid-based, pre-operation diet will include:

- Replacing your meals with fat-free protein shakes, vegetable juices, and fat-free broth

- A complete sugar-free diet – including drinks

- No alcohol and caffeine

- Everything has to be sipped slowly

Your diet plan before the operation will look something like this:

TIME	FOOD
8:00 AM	8oz protein smoothie
9:00 AM	8oz water
10:00 AM	8oz unsweetened juice or fat-free milk

11:00 AM	8oz decaffeinated tea or coffee
12:00 AM	8oz fat-free milk
1:00 PM	8oz protein smoothie
2:00 PM	8oz water
3:00 PM	8oz water
4:00 PM	8oz fat-free broth
5:00 PM	8oz water
6:00 PM	8oz unsweetened juice
7:00 PM	8oz water

8:00 PM	8oz protein smoothie

I have to point out again that it's extremely important to follow this type of diet strictly and obey all other rules your doctor tells you!

Gastric Bypass Surgery Risks

As I said earlier, this is a serious operation with some risks you have to keep in mind and discuss with your doctor before the procedure. First, you have to agree to some common risks related to any surgery, including gastric bypass. These risks include all the complications related to anesthesia and operation – allergic reactions to medicines, breathing problems, bleeding, blood cloths, and infections.

Risks that are typical for gastric bypass operation include: gastritis, heartburn, stomach and/or intestines injury during the procedure, stomach leaks, bad nutrition, vomiting, and stomach ulcers.

Make sure to fully understand these complications and follow your doctor's advice to reduce these risks to a minimum.

Diet After the Gastric Bypass Surgery

As I said earlier, gastric bypass surgery will make your stomach smaller which will automatically change the way your body handles the food you eat. Having your stomach smaller, your body will not absorb all the calories from the food you eat. In this, post operation period, your body will be recovering from the surgery and you will go through a healing process. Following the right diet plan will help you lose weight safely.

The first stage, right after the surgery, is the most critical one and will take some time for the body to get used to the new eating regimen. The exact length of this stage will be definitely determined by your physician. However, in this stage, you will have to follow a strict diet plan. Most foods will disrupt the healing process and even lead to vomiting. In the first few days, up to one week, after the surgery, your diet will be based on pure liquids. You should divide your meals into several smaller portions (2 to 3 ounces per portion) and drink slowly. It's the best option to drink smaller amounts of liquid every 1-2 hours. Also, make sure not to use a straw as they might disrupt your digestive system.

Liquids you can have during this stage are:

• Water

• Fat-free broth

• Fat-free milk

• Coconut water, sugar-free

• Unsweetened juice

• Decaffeinated tea or coffee

• Strained cream soup

Bellow you will find an example one-day meal plan to make it easier to understand this stage.

TIME	FOOD
8:00 AM	1oz water
9:00 AM	1-2oz water
10:00 AM	1-2oz unsweetened juice

TIME	FOOD
11:00 AM	1oz decaffeinated tea or coffee
12:00 AM	1oz coconut water
1:00 PM	1-2oz fat-free milk
2:00 PM	1-2oz water
3:00 PM	1-2oz water
4:00 PM	1oz fat-free broth
5:00 PM	1-2oz water
6:00 PM	1-2oz coconut water

TIME	FOOD
7:00 PM	1-2oz water
8:00 PM	1-2oz fat-free broth

Stage 1 Recipes

Delicious Broth Recipes

Bone broth is not some new diet trend but a powerful healing tool our ancestors have been using for thousands of years. It's one of the best things you can drink in the first stage of your recovery. Bone broth is loaded with calcium, magnesium, and phosphorus. It will boost up your entire organism and speed up the healing process. Make sure to prepare the broth without any extra fats and to drain out all the vegetable pieces before drinking it.

Making the Bone Broth

What bones to pick for what purpose (what part of what animal)

Just like with every other part of the animal, the first and the most important part of cooking your broth, is to choose the right bones. As I mentioned earlier, it is crucial to know where your bones came from. Healthy, grass-fed and organic bones will release the highest amounts of gelatin, vitamins, minerals, and flavor. Choose grass-fed beef bones, pasture-raised and free-range poultry, as well as wild-caught fish. Only these animals can produce all the healthy benefits of bone broth.

These types of bones that require an organic farming are sometimes challenging to find and can cost more. But they are definitely worth it – only these bones will provide the best flavor and nutrition. Bones that have high cartilage content, marrow, and gelatin are the best bones to include in your bone broth.

Regarding animal parts, there are a couple of things to learn before buying your bones. When it comes to beef bones, the best parts are: beef shank, oxtail, knucklebones, and feet. These bones have high concentrations of gelatin that will be released while cooking. Be creative and use every opportunity to create your bone broth. If you're preparing a nice stew with meat, why not use the bones for a nice broth that can stay in the freezer up to a month. The worst option is to let highly nutritive bones to go to waste.

In poultry like chicken and turkey, you can really use the entire carcass that is left after the roasting or frying. Chicken feet and even head are loaded with gelatin and different nutrients. Use every opportunity to prepare yourself a nice chicken broth.

When it comes to gelatin content, the best possible bones come from beef and pork. However, fish carcasses along with heads can be a beautiful basis for a delicious fish broth that can be used in so many different recipes.

Choosing the bone broth for cooking really depends on your taste. If you prefer a tender chicken flavor than start with high-quality chicken bones and prepare yourself a valuable broth that you can use for meals or drinks. Same goes for beef fans. However, you can be creative and combine several different types of bones – this will give you an interesting taste and extremely valuable broth.

The equipment

Almost all cooking appliances can be used to prepare a bone broth. As mentioned in the introduction part, bone broth is one of the oldest recipes known to mankind. This means that you won't have to buy some fancy and expensive machines to prepare this valuable food. All you need is a large, deep pot and you're probably good to go. This method, however, requires lots of responsibility and constant supervision which is not always practical. Leaving the stove on its own can cause disasters so make sure you're around all the time.

This, of course, doesn't mean you can't prepare your bone broth in a pressure or a slow cooker. In fact, cooking bones in a pressure cooker can give you a high-quality bone broth within a couple of hours and save you lots of time.

My personal favorite way of preparing a delicious bone broth is definitely a slow cooker. This appliance has both – the long cooking period that is the closest we can get to those nice old-fashioned recipes, but it also has the practical side. High-quality slow cookers don't require any special attention during cooking. You can simply plug in your device, set up the time, and leave. The machine will finish the process for you.

The Cooking Process

Just like every other recipe, cooking the bone broth does include some tips and tricks you have to master in order to prepare the best possible broth. When preparing your bone broth, there are a couple of things you need to keep in mind. First is the cooking time. As I mentioned earlier, no matter which appliance you choose to prepare your bone broth, it will take time. The most convenient way is to use the pressure cooker and reduce the cooking time. However, keep in mind that the more you cook your bones, the better your broth will be.

Another trick you will probably find useful is roasting the bones before cooking them. This way, your bones will have that superb roasted flavor and give your broth an entirely new dimension.

As for the mineral content in your broth, which is why you're preparing it in the first place, you need to know that soaking the bones will ensure that minerals will be pulled out of the bones into the broth. The best way is to soak cold bones with vinegar before cooking them. In order to soak the chicken bones, you will need two tablespoons of vinegar and one gallon of water. Beef bones, on the other hand, require more vinegar – half-cup for one gallon of water.

Now that you have prepared your bones, the cooking process will be easy. Start by adding vegetables, herbs, and spices into your broth. Some basic ingredients that are common in broths are onions, carrots, parsley, and celery stalk. However, keep in mind that parsley and celery leaves, along with other tender herbs and spices, won't require so much cooking. On the contrary, it will probably destroy their flavor and leave you without the specific aroma you're after. This is why you should be adding herbs and spices like parsley leaves, thyme, rosemary, fresh oregano, and other at the end of your cooking.

Basic Beef Broth

Ingredients:

4 lbs beef marrow bones

5 quarts water

1 tbsp lemon juice

1 bay leaf

Preparation:

Rinse and drain the bones.

In a large bowl, or a deep pot, combine water with lemon juice. Submerge bones in this mixture and soak for 30 minutes.

Transfer to a pressure cooker. Add one bay leaf and close the cooker's lid. Set the steam release handle and cook for 2 hours.

Drain and reserve the liquid.

Lamb Broth with Celery Roots

Ingredients:

4 lbs lamb marrow bones, raw

4 quarts water

2 large onions, peeled and sliced

2 large carrots, whole

2 medium-sized celery roots, whole

½ cup celery leaves, finely chopped

Preparation:

Place bones in your pressure cooker and add onions, celery roots, carrots, and salt. Pour in water and seal the lid. Cook for 3 hours.

Release the pressure and open the lid. Add finely chopped parsley and continue to cook for five more minutes – with the cooker's lid off.

Turn off the heat and drain the liquid.

You can prepare the recipe in a slow cooker. It will take 12-24 hours.

Chicken Broth with Spring Onions

Ingredients:

4 lbs chicken necks and backs

4 quarts water

1 cup spring onions, finely chopped

¼ tsp salt

1 tbsp apple cider vinegar

Preparation:

Place bones in a deep pot. Pour in the water, add salt and vinegar. Bring it to a boil and reduce the heat to low. Cover and simmer for 10 hours.

After ten hours add spring onions and bring it to a boil again. Cook for 15 more minutes. Drain the liquid and store.

You can reduce the cooking time by using a pressure cooker. It takes one hour to prepare this broth in a pressure cooker.

Basic Beef Broth with Bay Leaves

Ingredients:

5 lbs beef marrow bones

5 quarts water

1 tbsp red wine vinegar

5-6 bay leaves

1 tbsp salt

Preparation:

Combine water and red wine vinegar in a large pot. Soak the bones for one hour.

Transfer to a pressure cooker and add bay leaves and salt. Seal the lid and cook for 2-3 hours.

Allow the pressure to release naturally and open the lid. Strain out bones and store the broth.

Spring Fish Broth

Ingredients:

2 lbs sea bream, whole and cleaned

1 cup leeks, chopped

2 large carrots, sliced

1 medium-sized zucchini, chopped

1 medium-sized celery root, chopped

1 cup fresh celery leaves, chopped

3 tsp salt

1 tbsp fresh rosemary leaves, finely chopped

1 tbsp dried thyme

2 tbsp freshly squeezed lemon juice

3 quarts water

Preparation:

Rinse and clean the fish. Drain in a large colander and set aside.

Combine the ingredients in a deep pot. Bring it to a boil and reduce the heat to minimum.

Cook for 4-6 hours, stirring occasionally.

Remove from the heat and drain the liquid into containers. Store.

Lemon Ginger Broth

Ingredients:

2 lbs organic chicken breasts with skin (and any other parts such as necks and feet)

1 small ginger knob, about 1-inch thick

1 medium-sized onion, finely chopped

2 tbsp extra virgin olive oil

2 tbsp apple cider vinegar

1 tsp salt

1 tbsp fresh lemon juice

1 tsp freshly grated lemon zest

10 cups water

Preparation:

Preheat the oil in a deep pot over a medium-high temperature. Add the onions and stir-fry for about 3-5 minutes, or until translucent. Add chicken, lemon zest, and ginger. Cook for 10 minutes and then add water and vinegar. Bring it to a boil and then reduce the heat to low.

Cover with a lid and cook for at least 3 hours. Remove from the heat and strain the broth. Chop the meat parts such as breasts into small pieces and reserve for another use.

Cool the broth completely to a room temperature. Refrigerate overnight before using.

Chicken Mushroom Broth

Ingredients:

2 lbs chicken bones, (necks, backs, feet)

10 Shiitake mushrooms, stems removed and chopped

4 large carrots, cut into bite-sized pieces

2 medium-sized celery stalks, chopped

2 medium-sized leeks, chopped

5 garlic cloves, peeled

1 medium-sized onion, sliced

2 tbsp extra virgin olive oil

2 tsp turmeric, ground

1 tsp salt

Preparation:

Place the bones in a deep pot and add enough water to cover all. Cook for 2 hours on a low heat. Now, add mushrooms, carrots, leeks, garlic, onions, olive oil, and turmeric. Add more water to cover all again. Cook for 2 more hours on a low heat.

When done, remove from the heat and stir in the salt immediately. Let it cool completely to a room temperature. Strain the broth out of bones and vegetables.

Onion Bone Broth

Ingredients:

2 lbs beef marrow bones

1 cup apple cider vinegar

2 large onions, wedged

5 garlic cloves, peeled

1 large celery stalk, chopped

2 head baby Bok Choy, chopped

1 tsp salt

½ tsp black pepper, ground

Preparation:

Place the bones in a deep pot. Add apple cider vinegar and add enough water to cover all. Bring it to a boil and then reduce to a low heat. Cook for 2 hours.

Now, add onions, garlic, celery, Bok Choy, and kale. Add 3 cups of water and cook for 3 hours on low heat. Remove from the heat and stir in the salt and pepper immediately. Let it cool to a room temperature.

Strain out the bones and vegetables from the broth.

Fish Broth

Ingredients:

1 lb fish bones and heads, (eyes removed)

1 large onion, chopped

1 medium-sized celery stalk

1 medium-sized carrot, cut into strips

1 tsp black pepper

2 tbsp fresh parsley, finely chopped

9 cups of water

Preparation:

Pour the water in a large pot. Add the fish bones, onions, celery, and carrot. Bring it to a boil and then reduce the heat to low. Cook for 30 minutes.

Sprinkle with parsley and pepper. Give it a good stir and using a large wooden spoon, remove the foam from the top.

Strain the broth out of the fish bones. Let it cool to a room temperature.

Store the broth in a single-served air-tight container and refrigerate up to 2 days.

The broth can stay in the freezer up to 4 months.

Pork Thyme Broth

Ingredients:

4 lbs pork marrow bones

1 cup apple cider vinegar

1 whole lemon, juiced

2 tbsp fresh thyme, finely chopped

1 tbsp fresh coriander, chopped

¼ tsp cumin, ground

2 whole garlic cloves, peeled

1 medium-sized onion, wedged

1 tbsp fresh sage, roughly chopped

Preparation:

Place the bones in a deep pot. Add apple cider vinegar, lemon, and pour water enough to cover all. Bring it to a boil and then reduce the heat. Using a large slotted spoon, skim the foam from the surface.

Cook for 6 hours. 15 minutes before set, stir in the vegetables, herbs, and spices.

Remove from the heat and set aside to cool completely. Strain the broth and store it in an air-tight containers and refrigerate up to 7 days. Freeze up to 6 months.

Easy Juice Recipes

When you juice, the juicing machine extracts the juice from whole fruits or vegetables. The processing results in the same amount of vitamins and minerals, and it is perfect for the post operation stage. One cup of freshly squeezed, sugar-free juice will provide huge amounts of vitamins and minerals in just one glass and gently clean the entire gastro intestinal tract.

Tomato Juice

Ingredients:

3 large tomatoes

2 large carrots, sliced

2 celery stalks

1 large cucumber

1 bunch of fresh spinach

1 large bell pepper

Preparation:

Wash the tomatoes and place them in a bowl. Cut into small pieces and reserve the juices in a bowl while cutting. Set aside.

Wash the carrots and slice into a bowl with tomatoes.

Wash the celery and cucumber and chop into small pieces. add to the bowl.

Wash the bell pepper and cut in half. Remove the seeds and chop into small pieces.

Wash the spinach thoroughly and roughly chop it. Set aside.

Now, process tomatoes, carrots, celery, cucumber, spinach, and bell pepper in a juicer. Transfer to serving glasses.

Beet Pear Juice

Ingredients:

1 medium-sized beet, trimmed

1 large lemon, peeled

3 large pears

1 cup of fresh raspberries

Preparation:

Wash the beet and trim off the green ends. Chop into bite-sized pieces and place in a bowl.

Peel the lemon and cut it lengthwise. Set aside.

Wash the pears and remove the cores. Set aside.

Place the raspberries in a colander and wash under cold running water. Drain and set aside.

Now, process beets, lemon, pears, and raspberries in a juicer. Transfer to serving glasses and add few ice cubes.

Enjoy!

Chia Pepper Juice

Ingredients:

3 tbsp of chia seeds

1 large lemon, peeled

½ red bell pepper, seeded

½ yellow bell pepper, seeded

1 green apple, cored

Preparation:

Peel the lemon and cut lengthwise in half. Place it in a bowl and set aside.

Wash the bell pepper and cut in half. Remove the seeds and cut one-half of each in a bowl. Reserve the rest for some other juice.

Wash the apple and remove the core. Cut into bite-sized pieces and set aside.

Now, process lemon, bell peppers, and apple in a juicer. Transfer to serving glasses and stir in the chia seeds. Refrigerate for 15 minutes and stir again. Add some water to adjust the thickness, if needed.

Enjoy!

Apricot Grapefruit Juice

Ingredients:

1 large apricot, pitted

1 large grapefruit, peeled

1 cup of broccoli

1 large banana

Preparation:

Wash the apricot and cut in half. Remove the pit and cut into small pieces. Set aside.

Wash the grapefruit and cut into bite-sized pieces. Set aside.

Place the broccoli in a colander and wash under cold running water. Chop into small pieces and set aside.

Peel the banana and cut into small chunks. Set aside.

Now, process apricot, grapefruit, broccoli, and banana in a juicer. Transfer to serving glasses.

Ginger Butternut Squash Juice

Ingredients:

½ cup of butternut squash cubes

2 slices of fresh ginger

1 large red delicious apple, peeled and cored

1 large carrot

1 tbsp of fresh mint, finely chopped

1 large orange, peeled

1 tsp of pure coconut sugar

Preparation:

Peel the butternut squash and remove the seeds using a spoon. Cut into small cubes. Wash the apple and remove the core. Cut into bite-sized pieces and set aside.

Wash the carrot and cut into small slices. Set aside.

Peel the orange and divide into wedges. Set aside.

Peel the ginger slices and cut into small pieces. Set aside.

Combine mint and coconut sugar in a small bowl. Add about 2 tablespoons of water and let it stand for 5 minutes.

Now, process butternut squash, apple, carrot, and orange in a juicer.

Honeydew Melon Juice

Ingredients:

2 large honeydew melon wedges

5 tbsp of fresh mint

1 cup of avocado, peeled and pitted

1 large lime, peeled

Preparation:

Cut the honeydew melon lengthwise in half. Scoop out the seeds using a spoon. Cut the large wedges and peel them. Cut into small chunks and place in a bowl. Wrap the rest of the melon in a plastic foil and refrigerate.

Peel the avocado and cut in half. Remove the pit and cut into chunks. Add it to the bowl with melon and set aside.

Peel the lime and cut lengthwise in half. Set aside.

Wash the mint leaves and soak in water for 5 minutes.

Now, process honeydew melon, avocado, lime, and mint in a juicer. Serve.

Berry Beet Juice

Ingredients:

1 cup of blackberries

1 cup of blueberries

1 cup of fresh basil

1 large beet, trimmed

2 oz of coconut water

Preparation:

Combine blackberries and blueberries in a colander and wash under cold running water. Set aside.

Wash the beet and trim off the green ends. Chop into small pieces and set aside.

Wash the basil thoroughly and roughly chop it using hands.

Now, combine blackberries, blueberries, beet and basil in a juicer and process until juiced.

Transfer to serving glasses and stir in the coconut water.

Pomegranate Watermelon Juice

Ingredients:

1 cup of watermelon, peeled and seeded

1 large orange, peeled

1 cup of Romaine lettuce, shredded

1 cup of pomegranate seeds

Preparation:

Cut the watermelon lengthwise. For one cup, you will need about 1 large wedge. Peel and cut into chunks. Remove the seeds and set aside.

Cut the top of the pomegranate fruit using a sharp knife. Slice down to each of the white membranes inside of the fruit. Pop the seeds into a medium bowl.

Peel the orange and divide into wedges. Set aside.

Wash the lettuce thoroughly. Roughly chop it using hands and add set aside.

Now, process watermelon, orange, lettuce and pomegranate seeds in a juicer. Transfer to serving glasses and refrigerate before use.

Asparagus-Olive Oil Juice

Ingredients:

1 large green apple, cored

4 medium-sized asparagus spears, trimmed

1 large broccoli

3 large celery stalks

1 tbsp of extra-virgin olive oil

A handful of fresh parsley

Preparation:

Wash the apple and remove the core. Cut into bite-sized pieces and set aside.

Wash the asparagus and trim off the woody ends. Cut into small pieces and set aside.

Wash the celery stalks and broccoli. Chop into small pieces. Set aside.

Wash the parsley and finely chop it. Place it in a small bowl and add olive oil. Let it stand for 5 minutes.

Now, process apple, asparagus, broccoli, and celery in a juicer. Transfer to serving glasses and stir in the parsley and oil. You can sprinkle with some salt to taste if you like, but this is optional.

Serve immediately.

Green Kiwi Juice

Ingredients:

2 whole leeks, chopped

1 cup of Brussels sprouts, chopped

1 cup of parsley, chopped

2 whole kiwis, chopped

A handful of spinach, chopped

½ cup of water

Preparation:

Wash the leeks and chop into small pieces. Set aside.

Wash the Brussels sprouts and trim off the outer leaves. Cut in half and set aside.

Wash the parsley in a colander under cold running water and set aside.

Peel the kiwis and cut in half. Set aside.

Wash the spinach thoroughly and set aside.

Now, process leeks, Brussels sprouts, parsley, kiwis, and spinach in a juicer. Transfer to serving glasses and stir in the water.

Summer Guava Juice

Ingredients:

1 cup of pineapple chunks

1 whole guava, chopped

2 cups of chard, chopped

2 whole lemons, peeled

½ cup of coconut water, unsweetened

Preparation:

Cut the top of a pineapple and peel it using a sharp knife. Cut into small chunks. Reserve the rest of the pineapple in a refrigerator.

Wash the guava and cut into chunks. If you are using large fruit, reserve the rest for some other recipe in a refrigerator.

Wash the chard thoroughly under cold running water and set aside.

Peel the lemons and cut lengthwise in half. Set aside.

Now, process pineapple, guava, chard, and lemons in a juicer. Transfer to serving glasses and stir in the coconut water.

Turnip Artichoke Juice

Ingredients:

1 cup of turnip greens

1 large cucumber

1 large artichoke head

5 large asparagus spears

Preparation:

Wash the turnip greens and roughly chop it using hands. Set aside.

Wash the cucumber and cut into thick slices. Set aside.

Using a sharp knife, trim off the outer leave of the artichoke. Cut into small pieces and set aside.

Wash the asparagus spears and trim off the woody ends. Cut into small pieces and set aside.

Now, process turnip greens, cucumber, artichoke, and asparagus in a juicer.

Transfer to serving glasses and add few ice cubes before serving.

Grapefruit Kiwi Juice

Ingredients:

2 kiwis, peeled

1 cup of carrots, chopped

2 cups of green cabbage, shredded

1 whole grapefruit, peeled

1 tbsp of honey, raw

Preparation:

Peel the kiwis and cut in half. Set aside.

Wash the carrots and cut into small pieces. Set aside.

Wash the cabbage thoroughly and roughly chop it using hands.
Set aside.

Wash the grapefruit and cut into chunks. Set aside.

Now, process kiwis, carrots, cabbage, and grapefruit in a juicer.
Transfer to serving glasses and stir in the honey.

Add some ice cubes and serve immediately.

Cherry Juice

Ingredients:

1 cup of cherries, pitted

1 medium-sized banana

1 large cucumber

1 large carrot

Preparation:

Place the cherries in a colander and wash under cold running water. Remove the pits and set aside.

Peel the banana and cut into small chunks. Set aside.

Wash the cucumber and carrot. Chop into small pieces and set aside.

Now, process cherries, banana, cucumber, and carrot in a juicer.

Transfer to serving glasses and add some ice before serving.

Enjoy!

Bell Pepper Juice

Ingredients:

1 small red bell pepper, seeded

1 small green bell pepper, seeded

1 small yellow bell pepper, seeded

1 cup of broccoli

1 cup of fresh kale

Preparation:

Wash the bell peppers and cut in half. Remove the seeds and chop into small pieces. Set aside.

Wash the broccoli and kale in a colander under cold running water. Chop into small pieces and set aside.

Now, process peppers, broccoli, and kale in a juicer. Transfer to serving glasses and add a pinch of Cayenne pepper if you like it spicier. However, this is optional.

Serve immediately.

Stage Two After the Operation

After you've spent seven to ten days drinking pure liquids, your physician will give you the permission to enter the second post-surgery stage. This period usually lasts anywhere between 7-14 days, depending on your recovery speed. Now is the time to start eating moderate amounts of pureed proteins like mashed chicken or fish meat. Because of your small stomach size, you will start with a couple of small meals per day – 60-70 grams of proteins and 67 ounces of liquids per day. However, you should still be avoiding simple carbs, sugars, caffeinated and carbonated beverages. The best food choices are:

- protein smoothies

- egg whites

- non-fat cheese

- non-fat yogurts

- mashed vegetables

- mashed beans

- lean ground meat

- blended fish and chicken meat

Besides these foods, you can include all foods from the stage one – drink them as they are or use them to prepare smoothies. However, it's very important to point out that you shouldn't eat and drink at the same time. Wait for about 30 minutes to 1 hour after each meal to drink something. Learn to listen carefully listen to your organism. If you feel like you're still sensitive to certain foods, it's better to avoid them.

Bellow, you will find one-day sample meal plan:

TIME	FOOD
8:00 AM	1oz water
9:00 AM	5oz smoothie
10:00 AM	2 egg whites
11:00 AM	1oz decaffeinated tea or coffee
12:00 AM	5oz mashed chicken meat
1:00 PM	8oz fat-free milk
2:00 PM	1-2oz water
3:00 PM	1-2oz water
4:00 PM	5oz smoothie

TIME	FOOD
5:00 PM	1-2oz water
6:00 PM	8oz coconut water
7:00 PM	1-2oz water
8:00 PM	8oz fat-free broth

Stage 2 Recipes

Pureed Beef Cabbage Stew

Ingredients:

2 lbs beef marrow bones

2 cups green cabbage, shredded

1 medium-sized onion, sliced

2 large carrots, sliced

2 tbsp fresh parsley, finely chopped

1 tsp fresh rosemary, minced

1 tbsp tomato paste

1 tsp salt

2 tbsp apple cider vinegar

Preparation:

Wash and prepare the vegetables.

Place the bones in a deep pot. Add apple cider vinegar and then pour water enough to cover all the bones. Let it soak at least an hour.

Now, heat up a large pot over a medium temperature. Add all the vegetables and add more water if needed. Cook for 2 hours. You can reduce the cooking time if you place the bones in a pressure cooker. 40 minutes will be enough to prepare a broth.

Remove from the heat and drain the liquid. Transfer to a pot along with the remaining ingredients. Cook for 45 minutes, over medium heat.

Remove from the heat and transfer to a food processor. Blend until smooth.

Tomato Rib Soup

Ingredients:

2 lbs short ribs

2 lbs of medium-sized tomatoes, diced

1 cup of white beans, pre-cooked

1 cup of vegetable broth, fat-free

2 tbsp of fresh parsley, finely chopped

Preparation:

Place the bones in a deep pot. Add water enough to cover all the bones. Cook for 3 hours on a low heat. Remove from the heat and remove the bones from the pot. Set aside.

Transfer to a deep pot along with other ingredients. Reduce the heat to low and cook for 45 minutes, stirring occasionally.

Transfer to blender or a food processor and pulse until smooth.

Brussels Sprouts Puree

Ingredients:

1lb fresh brussel sprouts, halved

7 oz fresh baby spinach, torn

1 cup skim milk

3 tbsp Greek yogurt, fat-free

1 tbsp of fresh celery, finely chopped

Instructions:

Place brussels sprouts in a deep, heavy-bottomed pot. Pour enough water to cover and bring it to a boil. Cook until fork tender.

Now add spinach and continue to cook for 3 more minutes. Remove from the heat and drain. Transfer to a food processor along with other ingredients. Add one cup of fat-free broth and pulse to combine.

Serve.

Lamb Broth with Pumpkin

Ingredients:

2 lbs lamb marrow bones

1 lbs pumpkin, chopped

1 large onion, peeled and finely chopped

1 tbsp ground turmeric

A handful fresh parsley

Preparation:

Place the bones in a deep pot. Add water enough to cover all the bones. Simmer for 1 hour on a medium-low heat. Set aside.

Place pumpkin, turmeric, bones, and broth in a large pot. Bring it to a boil and reduce the heat to medium. Continue to cook for 15 minutes, stirring occasionally.

Remove from the heat and transfer to blender. Pulse until smooth.

Vegetable Chicken Broth

Ingredients:

2 lbs chicken necks and backs

1 cup fresh broccoli, chopped

1 cup artichoke, chopped

½ cup green peas

1 cup cherry tomatoes, halved

1 medium-sized celery stalk, chopped

½ cup fresh dill, chopped

1 small onion, sliced

1 medium-sized carrot, sliced

6 cups water

1 tbsp apple cider vinegar

Preparation:

In a deep pot, place the chicken necks and backs. Add vinegar and enough water to cover all. Cook for 2 hours on a low heat.

Wash and prepare the vegetables.

Preheat the oil in a deep pot over a low temperature. Add all vegetables and stir-fry for about 3-5 minutes.

Now, add about 6 cups of water and bring it to a boil. Cover with a lid and simmer for about an hour. Remove from the heat and set aside to cool for a while.

Using a large colander, drain the broth in a separated pot. You can use the broth for a meal preparation, or simply store it in the freezer up to 1 month.

Homemade Chicken Soup

Ingredients:

1 lb chicken meat

4 cups chicken broth

A handful fresh parsley

1 tsp salt

¼ tsp freshly ground black pepper

Preparation:

For this recipe, I always try to find an organic chicken. They are much tastier and better for a homemade soup. Use both, dark and white pieces and rinse well under the running water. Pat dry with a kitchen paper and place on a clean work surface.

Using a sharp cutting knife, cut the chicken into bite-sized pieces. Sprinkle with salt and place in a deep pot. If using organic chicken, be careful not to add extra fat..

Pour in the chicken broth and cover with the lid. Cook for 20 minutes and then remove the lid.

Remove from the heat and drain. Place the meat in a food processor and pulse until smooth.

Combine with broth again and serve.

Creamy Chicken Broth and Asparagus Soup

Ingredients:

2 lbs fresh wild asparagus, trimmed

2 small onions, peeled and finely chopped

1 cup Greek yogurt, fat-free

4 cups vegetable broth

1 tbsp fresh thyme, finely chopped

Preparation:

Rinse and drain asparagus. Trim off the woody ends and cut into one inch-thick pieces. Set aside.

Place in a large, heavy-bottomed pot. Pour in enough water to cover and bring it to a boil. Cook until fork-tender. Drain the asparagus but reserve the liquid. Mash with a potato masher and combine with broth again.

Stir in Greek yogurt and fresh thyme. Cook for five more minutes.

Broccoli and Cottage Cheese Puree

Ingredients:

10oz cottage cheese

1 cup broccoli, finely chopped

½ cup skim milk

4 cups beef broth, fat-free

1 tbsp parsley, finely chopped

Preparation:

Wash the broccoli and trim off the outer leaves. Slice and place in a deep pot. Add beef broth and cook until fork tender.

Transfer broccoli to a food processor and add milk, cottage cheese, and parsley. Pulse until smooth.

Serve.

Pureed Mackerel Fillets with Beans

Ingredients:

7 oz mackerel fillets

½ cup kidney beans, pre-cooked

1 lb fresh tomatoes, peeled and roughly chopped

4 cups fish broth

¼ tsp salt

1 tsp fresh rosemary, finely chopped

Preparation:

Rinse the fillets and drain in a large colander. Sprinkle with salt and set aside.

Heat up a non-stick, heavy-bottomed pot over medium heat. Add tomatoes and rosemary. Stir fry until soft. Now add the remaining ingredients and cook for 25 minutes, stirring occasionally.

Remove from the heat and transfer to a blender. Pulse until smooth.

Sour Cabbage Beef Broth

Ingredients:

2 lbs beef marrow bones

1 cup sauerkraut, shredded

1 cup apple cider vinegar

2 medium-sized carrots, sliced

1 medium-sized onion, wedged

1 cup tomatoes, diced

1 tsp salt

Preparation:

Place the bones in a deep pot. Add vinegar and pour water enough to cover all. Cook for 2 hours and then add sauerkraut, carrots, onions, and tomatoes.

Again, pour water enough to cover all, and then add 2 cups more. Bring it to a boil and then reduce the heat to low. Cook for 3 hours. Just before set, sprinkle with some dried thyme and sage. However, it is optional.

Remove from the heat and set aside to cool completely to a room temperature.

Strain out the bones and vegetables from the broth using a colander. Stir in some salt.

Store the broth in airtight container up to 7 days, or in a freezer up to 6 months.

Lean Cauliflower Chicken Broth

Ingredients:

2 lbs chicken backs, leftover bones, and skin

1 cup cauliflower, chopped

1 medium-sized onion, sliced

1 cup broccoli, chopped

2 medium-sized carrots, sliced

2 tbsp fresh parsley, finely chopped

1 tsp salt

1 tsp black pepper

Preparation:

Place the chicken parts in a deep pot. Add cauliflower, broccoli, carrots, and onions. Pour water enough to cover all the ingredients.

Sprinkle with salt and pepper and bring it to a boil. Reduce the heat to low and simmer for at least 4 hours. Using a wooden spatula, remove the foam from the surface while cooking.

Remove the pot from the heat. Remove the ingredients and gently strain the broth to an airtight containers or jars.

Store the broth in the freezer and use up to 1 month. However, if you want to have a broth for a longer period, than cook for an extra 2 hours, so it could stay up to 5-6 months.

Red Bell Pepper Beef Broth

Ingredients:

2 lbs beef knuckle bones

2 large red bell peppers, seeds removed and cut into rings

1 cup fresh cabbage, shredded

1 medium-sized onion, wedged

1 tsp salt

Preparation:

Place the bones in a deep pot. Add water enough to cover all and bring it to a boil. Reduce the heat to low and cook for 2 hours. Using a large slotted spoon, remove the foam from the surface from time to time.

Now, add prepared vegetables and season with salt. Cook for 2 more hours. Remove from the heat and strain out the broth from the bones and vegetables.

Pick up the pepper rings and place in a food processor. Pulse until smooth and serve with broth.

Garlic Chicken Broth

Ingredients:

1 whole chicken

2 medium-sized carrots, cut into chunks

1 small celery stalk, chopped

1 medium-sized onion, wedged

2 tbsp fresh parsley, finely chopped

2 garlic cloves, whole

½ tsp dried thyme, ground

Preparation:

Place the chicken in a large pot. Add enough water to cover the chicken. Bring it to a boil and then reduce the heat to low. Remove the foam from the surface using a large slotted spoon. Cook for 1 hour, turning the chicken once.

Remove from the heat and set aside to cool for a while. Now, transfer the chicken to a clean working wooden surface. Remove the meat and use for some other recipe.

Return the skin and bones to the pot in the same water. Add all the remaining ingredients and cook for 3 more hours over low heat.

Remove from the heat and strain the broth using a large colander. Let it cool completely and refrigerate. Use up to 3 days.

Beef Broth with Carrots

Ingredients:

2 lbs beef marrow bones, knuckle bones, and ribs

3 medium-sized carrots, peeled

1 medium-sized onion, peeled

2 parsley sprigs

1 tsp salt

Preparation:

Combine all ingredients in a deep pot. Add water enough to cover all ingredients and bring it to a boil. Reduce the heat to low and simmer for 2 hours.

Using a large slotted spoon, skim the foam out of the surface of the broth.

Remove from the heat and strain out the bones and vegetables. Pick up the carrots and return to the pot. Set aside to cool and mash the carrots with a potato masher. Stir well and serve.

Vitamin Boosting Chicken Broth

Ingredients:

4 lbs of chicken bones (backs, heads, wings, legs, etc.)

1 whole lemon, juiced

1 tsp ginger, ground

1 tsp salt

1 tsp peppercorn

Preparation:

Place the chicken bones in a deep pot. Add water enough to cover all. Bring it to a boil and then reduce the heat to low. Make sure to skim the foam from the surface.

Cook for 4 hours. When almost done, stir in the lemon juice, ginger, salt, and peppercorn. Cook for 15 minutes more and remove from the heat. Set aside to cool to a room temperature.

Strain the broth to into a large bowl. Store the broth in the air-tight jars and refrigerate up to 6-7 days, or freeze up to 6 months.

Blueberry-Almond Smoothie

Ingredients:

1 cup of fresh blueberries

¼ cup of toasted almonds

½ cup of Greek yogurt, fat-free

1 cup of almond milk

Preparation:

Using a large colander, rinse the blueberries under cold running water. Set aside.

Now, combine blueberries, toasted almonds, Greek yogurt, and almond milk in a food processor or a blender.

Process until well combined and creamy. Transfer to a serving glass and garnish with fresh mint. However, this is optional.

Serve immediately.

Pear Smoothie

Ingredients:

1 glass of skim milk, fat-free

¼ tsp of cinnamon, ground

1 medium-sized pear, roughly chopped

½ cup of fresh grapes

1 tbsp of flaxseed

Preparation:

Wash the pear and cut lengthwise in half. Using a sharp paring knife, remove the core. Cut into bite-sized pieces and set aside.

Rinse the grapes under cold running water and remove the stems. Set aside.

Now, combine pear, milk, ground cinnamon, grapes, and flaxseeds in a food processor or a blender. Process until smooth and creamy. Transfer to a serving glass and serve immediately.

Enjoy!

Vegetable Smoothie

Ingredients:

1 cup of cooked broccoli

1 cup baby spinach, chopped

½ cup of yogurt, fat-free

1 cup coconut water, sugar-free

1 tsp mint extract

Preparation:

Wash the broccoli and remove the outer leaves. Cut into bite-sized pieces and fill the measuring cup. Reserve the rest in the refrigerator.

Place the broccoli in a heavy-bottomed pot. Add water enough to cover and bring it to a boil. You can add a pinch of salt, but it's optional. Reduce the heat to low and cook for 2 minutes. Remove from the heat and drain well. Set aside to cool completely.

Rinse the baby spinach leaves under cold running water. Slightly drain and chop into small pieces.

Now, combine previously prepared broccoli, yogurt, coconut water, and mint extract in a food processor or a blender. Pulse until well incorporated and creamy.

Transfer to serving glasses and serve immediately.

Berry Blast Smoothie

Ingredients:

1 cup of mixed blueberries, raspberries, blackberries and strawberries

½ cup of chopped baby spinach

½ cup of coconut water, unsweetened

1 cup water

¼ tsp of ginger, ground

A handful of fresh mint leaves

Preparation:

Combine all berries in a large colander and rinse under cold running water. Make sure to remove the strawberry stems, if any.

Rinse the spinach under cold running water and drain in a large colander.

Now, combine all berries, spinach, coconut water, water, ginger and mint in a blender. Process until well combined and smooth.

Transfer to serving glasses and top with more berries for decoration. However, it's optional.

Serve immediately.

Mellon Strawberry Puree

Ingredients:

¼ cup of fresh strawberries, cut into bite-sized pieces

¼ of banana, thinly sliced

1 wedge of melon

½ tsp of cinnamon, ground

¼ cup of avocado, chopped

Preparation:

Wash the strawberries under cold running water and remove the stems. Cut into bite-sized pieces and set aside.

Peel the banana and cut into thin slices. Fill the measuring cup and reserve the rest for later.

Cut the melon lengthwise in half. Scoop out the seeds using a spoon. Cut one large wedge and peel it. Cut into small chunks and place in a bowl. Wrap the rest of the melon in a plastic foil and refrigerate.

Peel the avocado and cut lengthwise in half. Remove the pit and cut into bite-sized pieces. Fill the measuring cup and reserve the rest in the refrigerator.

Now, combine strawberries, banana, melon, cinnamon, and avocado in a food processor or a blender. Process until well combined and transfer to serving glasses.

Serve immediately.

Strawberry Smoothie

Ingredients:

½ cup of strawberries, cut into bite-sized pieces

¼ cup of fresh blueberries

1 cup of milk, fat-free

½ tsp of cinnamon, ground

Preparation:

Place the strawberries in a colander and wash under cold running water. Rinse well and drain. Remove the stems and cut into small pieces. Fill the measuring cup and reserve the rest for later. Set aside.

Rinse the blueberries in a colander and slightly drain. Set aside.

Now, combine strawberries, blueberries, milk, and cinnamon in a blender or a food processor. Process until well combined and transfer to a serving glass.

Garnish with some fresh mint or berries for some extra taste and serve immediately.

Vanilla Smoothie

Ingredients:

1 cup milk, fat-free

½ cup water

½ cup fresh strawberries, cut into bite-sized pieces

¼ cup fresh cranberries

1 tsp pure vanilla extract, sugar-free

¼ tsp ground cinnamon

Preparation:

Combine milk and water in a small, heavy-bottomed pot over a medium-high temperature. Bring it to a boil and then reduce the heat to low. Add minced vanilla and vanilla extract. Stir well and let it simmer for about a minute. Remove from the heath and allow it to cool completely.

Meanwhile, combine strawberries and cranberries in a large colander. Wash under cold running water and drain . Remove the strawberry stems and cut into bite-sized pieces.

Now, combine milk-vanilla mixture, strawberries, cranberries, and cinnamon in a food processor or a blender. Process until nicely combined and serve immediately.

Goji Berries Puree

Ingredients:

1 cup milk, fat-free

1 small Granny Smith's apple, cored and chopped

1 tbsp Greek yogurt, fat-free

1 banana, chopped

¼ cup goji berries

1 tsp fresh mint leaves

Preparation:

Wash the apple and cut lengthwise in half. Remove the core and chop into small pieces. Set aside.

Peel the banana and chop into small chunks. Set aside.

now, combine milk, apple, Greek yogurt, banana, goji berries, and mint leaves in a blender or a food processor. Pulse until nicely combined and smooth.

Transfer to serving glasses and top with some extra goji berries before serving.

Coffee Smoothie

Ingredients:

1 cup of unsweetened chilled coffee, decaf

1 cup of milk, fat-free

1 tsp pure vanilla extract, sugar-free

1 tbsp Greek yogurt

¼ tsp cinnamon, ground

Preparation:

Combine all the ingredients in a blender. Mix well for about 30 seconds. Transfer to a serving glass or a cup and serve immediately.

Flax Seed Apple smoothie

Ingredients:

½ medium-sized Alkmene apple, peeled and cut into bite-sized pieces

1 cup of baby spinach, finely chopped

1 cup of freshly squeezed orange juice, sugar-free

2 tbsp of flax seeds

Preparation:

Wash and peel the apple. Cut lengthwise in half and remove the core. Reserve one half in the refrigerator for some other smoothie. Cut into bite-sized pieces and set aside.

Rinse the baby spinach thoroughly under cold running water. Slightly drain and finely chop it. Set aside.

Now, combine apple, baby spinach, orange juice, and flax seeds in a food processor or a blender. Pulse until nicely combined.

Transfer to serving glasses and serve immediately.

Stage Three After the Surgery

After a couple of weeks of drinking liquids and eating pureed foods, your doctor will allow you to slowly start eating soft foods. In this stage, your diet will be based on small, tender, and easily chewed pieces of meat, cooked vegetables, and fruit. Make sure to eat lean parts of meat and not to add extra fats or sugar into your meals. This phase has one basic rule – overcooked is always better! Basically, make sure to cook properly your food and to finely chop it before eating. Unlike previous two, this phase is diverse and you can eat lots of foods you weren't allowed before.

Foods allowed in this stage:

- Lean chicken

- Lean turkey

- Fish

- Vegetables

- Fruits

- Cottage cheese, fat-free

- Tofu

- Yogurt, fat-free

Bellow you will find one-day meal plan:

TIME	FOOD
8:00 AM	4oz water
9:00 AM	3 scrambled whites
10:00 AM	8oz skim milk
11:00 AM	4oz decaffeinated tea or coffee
12:00 AM	2oz cooked chicken meat
1:00 PM	1 banana, mashed
2:00 PM	8oz water
3:00 PM	8oz chicken broth

TIME	FOOD
4:00 PM	5oz smoothie
5:00 PM	8oz water
6:00 PM	2oz tuna
7:00 PM	1-2oz water
8:00 PM	8oz fat-free broth

Stage 3 Recipes

Baked Apples

Ingredients:

2 medium-sized Honeycrisp apples

¼ cup freshly squeezed lemon juice

½ tsp cinnamon, ground

Preparation:

Preheat the oven to 375 degrees F.

Wash the apples, cut in half and remove the seeds. Combine the lemon juice with ground cinnamon and mix well. Spread this mixture over the apple using a kitchen brush.

Place the apple upright in a dish. Bake for about an hour, until the apple is soft.

Serve with one teaspoon of manuka honey or blackstrap molasses.

Greek Yogurt with Peach

Ingredients:

1 cup Greek yogurt

1 tsp coconut oil, melted

1 tsp coconut nectar

1 peach, finely chopped

½ cup walnuts, whole

Preparation:

Combine Greek yogurt with coconut oil and coconut nectar. Whisk well and pour into a serving glass. Top with walnuts and chopped peach.

Refrigerate for 15 minutes before serving.

Fruit Puree with Chia Seeds

Ingredients:

2 medium-sized plums, sliced

2 medium-sized figs, sliced

½ Alkmene apple, chopped into bite-sized pieces

1 tbsp of pumpkin seeds

1 tbsp of chia seeds

½ cup Greek yogurt

Preparation:

Wash the plums and cut lengthwise in half. Remove the pits and cut into bite-sized pieces. Set aside.

Wash the figs and slice into thin slices. Set aside.

Wash the apple and cut lengthwise in half. Remove the core and chop into bite-sized pieces. Set aside.

Now, place the fruit in a medium bowl. Add figs and toss to combine. Sprinkle with pumpkin seeds and chia seeds. Transfer all a food processor or a blender. Process until well combined and transfer to a serving bowl. Stir in the Greek yogurt and sprinkle with some fresh mint. However, it's optional.

Serve cold.

Braised Swiss Chard

Ingredients:

1 lb of Swiss chard, torn (keep the stems)

2 medium-sized potatoes, finely chopped

1 small onion, chopped

2 garlic cloves, finely chopped

1 tsp of salt

¼ tsp of black pepper, ground

Preparation:

Wash the Swiss chard thoroughly under cold running water. Torn with hands and set aside.

Place Swiss chard in a large, heavy-bottomed pot. Add enough water to cover and bring it to a boil. Briefly cook, for about 3 minutes until greens are tender. Drain in a colander and set aside.

Preheat a large, non-stick skillet over a medium-high temperature. Add onions and garlic and stir-fry for about 3-4 minutes, or until translucent. Add potatoes and 1 cup of water. Bring it to a boil and reduce the heat to low. Cook for 15 minutes, or until water evaporates. Add Swiss chard and sprinkle with some salt and pepper. Cook for 2 more minutes and then remove from the heat.

Serve.

Lean Chicken Okra with Jerusalem Artichokes

Ingredients:

7oz chicken breast, boneless and skinless

1 lb okra, rinsed and trimmed

3 large Jerusalem artichokes, whole

2 medium-sized tomatoes, halved

2-3 fresh cauliflower florets

2 cups of vegetable broth

A handful of fresh broccoli

1 tsp of Himalayan salt

Preparation:

Cut each okra pod in half lengthwise and place in a deep pot. Add tomato halves, Jerusalem artichokes, cauliflower florets, a handful of fresh broccoli. Top with meat and season with salt. Pour in two cups of vegetable broth and give it a good stir.

Bring it to a boil and reduce the heat to medium. Cook for one hour, stirring occasionally.

Remove from the heat and finely chop the meat and vegetables. Jerusalem artichokes should be tender enough to mash them with a potato masher.

Optionally, transfer the entire stew to a food processor and blend until smooth.

Wild Salmon with Greens

Ingredients:

1 lb of wild salmon filets, boneless and skinless

1 lb of fresh spinach, torn

2 garlic cloves, finely chopped

2 tbsp of lemon juice

1 tbsp of fresh rosemary, chopped

1 tsp of sea salt

3 cups fish stock, fat-free

Preparation:

Rinse the meat and sprinkle with sea salt. Place at the bottom of a deep pot. Drizzle with lemon juice and add garlic, and rosemary. Pour in the fish stock and bring it to a boil.

Cook until completely tender, for 20-25 minutes, over medium heat. Remove from the heat and finely chop. Set aside.

Briefly boil the spinach, for 3 minutes. Drain and serve with combine with chopped salmon fillet. Toss well before serving.

Whole Chicken and Vegetable Stew

Ingredients:

1 whole chicken, 3 lbs

10 oz of fresh broccoli

7 oz cauliflower florets

1 large onion, peeled and finely chopped

1 large potato, peeled and finely chopped

3 medium-sized carrots, finely chopped

1 large tomato, finely chopped

A handful of yellow wax beans, finely chopped

A handful of fresh parsley, finely chopped

6 cups chicken broth

Preparation:

Clean the chicken and wash throughly under cold running water. Pat dry with a kitchen towel and place at the bottom of a deep pot.

Add vegetables and finely chopped parsley. Pour in 6 cups of chicken broth and bring it to a boil.

Reduce the heat and simmer for 3 hours.

Remove from the heat and finely chop the meat before serving.

Sour Zucchini Stew

Ingredients:

4 medium-sized zucchini, peeled and sliced

1 large eggplant, peeled and chopped

3 medium-sized red bell peppers, thinly sliced

½ cup fresh tomato juice

2 tsp of fresh thyme

½ tsp of salt

Preparation:

Peel the zucchinis and slice them into thin slices. Set aside.

Peel the eggplant and cut into small chunks. Set aside.

Wash the bell peppers and cut lengthwise in half. Scoop out the seeds and cut into thin slices. Set aside.

Preheat a large, non-stick skillet over a medium-high heat. Add sliced zucchini and eggplant, red bell peppers, and tomato juice. Stir well and season with some salt and thyme. Give it a good stir and pour about ½ cup of water. Bring it to a boil and then reduce the heat to low. Cover with a lid and cook for 25-30 minutes. Stir occasionally.

Cold Cauliflower Salad

Ingredients:

7 oz cauliflower florets, finely chopped

7oz broccoli, finely chopped

½ cup freshly squeezed orange juice, sugar-free

1 tsp fresh mint leaves, finely chopped

¼ tsp of salt

5 cups vegetable broth

Preparation:

Combine cauliflower and broccoli in a large colander. Rinse well under cold running water and drain. Cut into bite-sized pieces.

Place the vegetables in a heavy-bottomed pot. Pour in vegetable broth and season with salt and fresh mint.

Bring it to a boil and cook until completely tender. Drain and drizzle with orange juice.

Chill completely before serving.

Chicken Wings and Green Peppers Stew

Ingredients:

1 lb chicken breast, boneless and skinless

2 large potatoes, peeled and finely chopped

5 large green bell peppers, finely chopped

2 small carrots, finely chopped

2 ½ cups of chicken broth

1 large tomato, roughly chopped

A handful of fresh parsley, finely chopped

½ tsp of salt

Preparation:

Rinse the chicken breast under cold running water. Pat-dry with a kitchen paper. Cut into bite-sized pieces and set aside.

Heat up a large, non-stick skillet. Add vegetables and stir-fry for a couple of minutes, stirring constantly. Transfer to a deep pot and add chicken breast, chicken broth, parsley, and salt.

Bring it to a boil and give it a good stir. Reduce the heat to medium and simmer for 2 hours, stirring constantly.

Remove from the heat and set aside to cool for a while. Top with some extra parsley for some extra taste. However, it's optional.

Braised Greens with Fresh Mint

Ingredients:

3.5 oz fresh chicory, torn

3.5 oz wild asparagus, finely chopped

3.5 oz Swiss chard, torn

A handful of fresh mint, chopped

A handful of rocket salad, torn

1 garlic clove, crushed

1 tsp of salt

¼ cup of fresh lemon juice

1 tbsp olive oil

Preparation:

Combine chicory, asparagus, Swiss chard, mint, and rocket salad in a large colander. Rinse well and drain. Chop the greens into small pieces. Cut the wooden ends of the asparagus and finely chop it.

Fill a large pot with salted water and add greens. Bring it to a boil and cook for 2-3 minutes. Remove from the heat and drain.

Grease a medium-sized skillet with olive oil. Add crushed garlic and stir-fry for 2-3 minutes. Now, add the greens, salt, pepper, and about half of the lemon juice. Stir-fry the greens for five more minutes.

Remove from the heat. Season with more lemon juice and serve.

Chicken Pudding with Artichoke Hearts

Ingredients:

1 lb dark and white chicken meat, cooked

2 artichokes

1 lemon, juiced

1 handful of fresh parsley leaves

1 tsp of pink Himalayan salt

Preparation:

If possible, use organic chicken meat (breast and thighs). Thoroughly rinse the meat and pat dry with a kitchen paper. Using a sharp cutting knife, cut the meat into smaller pieces and remove the bones.

Heat the saute pan over medium-high heat. Turn the heat down to medium and add the meat. Cook for about one minute to get it a little golden one one side. Then flip each piece, cover the pan with a thigh fitting lid and turn the heat to low. Cook for ten minutes without removing the lid. This will poach your meat from the inside out in its own juices. This is why it's important that the lid stays on all the time.

Now turn off the heat and let it sit for another ten minutes. It has to stay covered the whole time. Take the lid off the pan and set aside allowing the meat to cool for a while.

Meanwhile, prepare the artichoke. Cut the lemon into halves and squeeze the juice in a small bowl. Divide the juice in half and set aside.

Using a sharp paring knife, trim off the outer leaves until you reach the yellow and soft ones. Trim off the green outer skin around the artichoke base and stem. Make sure to remove the 'hairs' around the artichoke heart. They are inedible so simply throw them away. Cut artichoke into half-inch pieces. Rub with half of the lemon juice and place in a heavy-bottomed pot. Add enough water to cover and cook until completely fork-tender. Remove from the heat and drain. Chill for a while (to a room temperature). I like to cut each piece into thin strips, but this is optional.

Now combine artichoke with chicken meat in a large bowl. Stir in salt and the remaining lemon juice. Serve.

Spinach and Chicken Soup

Ingredients:

1 lb chicken breast, boneless and skinless, chopped into bite-sized pieces

7 oz spinach, torn

2 medium-sized onions, finely chopped

4 cups chicken broth

1 tbsp Italian seasoning mix

Preparation:

Rinse well the meat and rub with Italian seasoning mix. Place in a deep pot and add broth. Bring it to a boil and cook for 45 minutes. Remove from the heat and set aside.

Meanwhile, rinse the spinach thoroughly under cold running water. Drain well and torn with hands into small pieces. Set aside.

Peel the onions and finely chop it. Set aside.

Preheat a large, non-stick skillet over medium heat. Add onions and stir-fry for five minutes. Add spinach and continue to cook for five more minutes.

Finally, add meat, broth, and one more cup of water. Bring it to a boil and remove from the heat.

Serve immediately.

Creamy Pea Puree

Ingredients:

1 cup of cooked peas

Large handful of spinach, torn

1 small onion, finely chopped

1 cup skim milk

2 tbsp of tahini

1 garlic clove, crushed

½ salt

Preparation:

Place the peas in a heavy-bottomed pot. Add about three cups of water and bring it to a boil. Cook for 15 minutes, or until soft. Remove from the heat and drain well. Set aside to cool.

Wash the spinach thoroughly under cold running water. Drain and torn with hands into small pieces. Set aside.

Peel the onion and finely chop it. Set aside.

Now, combine previously cooked peas, spinach, onion, milk, tahini, garlic, and salt in a food processor. Process until well pureed and creamy. Transfer to a serving bowl and serve immediately.

Creamy Broccoli Casserole

Ingredients:

2 large broccoli crowns, chopped

7 oz Brussels sprouts, halved

4 cups vegetable broth

2 small onions, finely chopped

1 cup of Greek yogurt, fat-free

2 tsp dry thyme

½ tsp salt

Preparation:

Preheat the oven to 400 degrees.

Wash the broccoli crowns under cold running water and cut into bite-sized pieces. Set aside.

Wash the Brussels sprouts and trim off the outer wilted layers. Cut each sprout in half and set aside.

In a large saucepan, combine vegetable broth with thyme and salt. Bring it to a boil and remove from the heat.

Heat up a large, non-stick skillet. Add onions and stir-fry for 2-3 minutes, or until translucent. Now add chopped broccoli and brussel sprouts. Pour in half of the broth and cook for ten minutes.

Stir in Greek yogurt and transfer to a shallow casserole dish.

Bake for about 20 minutes, or until the top is lightly charred and crisp.

Serve!

Creamy Button Mushroom Soup

Ingredients:

1lb fresh button mushrooms, thinly sliced

2 garlic cloves, crushed

Few sprigs of fresh thyme, finely chopped

1 medium-sized onion, finely chopped

5 cups vegetable broth

½ tsp of sea salt

1 tbsp of fresh parsley, finely chopped

Preparation:

Wash the mushrooms thoroughly under cold running water. Remove the stems cut into thin slices. Set aside.

Heat up a large, non-stick skillet, over medium-high heat. Add onion, garlic and stir-fry for 2-3 minutes, stirring constantly.

Transfer the onions to a heavy-bottomed pan. Add the mushrooms, thyme, salt, and vegetable broth. Cook for 10 minutes over medium heat.

Top with finely chopped parsley before serving.

The Final Phase of Your Post Operation Recovery

After going through three phases of your recovery journey, it is time to start eating some solid foods. This phase will start only when your body is able to tolerate all the food from the stage 3. However, you have to keep in mind that you're still not able to digest large pieces of food. Start very slowly and chop the foods before you eat them. A good advice is to write down what you eat. This way you can experiment with your body and find out what foods you can tolerate. This is the stage where you can try to eat everything, but in moderate amounts. Remember, your body is still adjusting to a new diet regimen. It will take time for you to fully recover. So be patient.

There are some basic rules you will have to follow in order to help your body heal and lose some weight in a natural and healthy way.

Your daily menu has to be divided between several small portions of food. The best plan is to eat 3 major meals per day and a couple of small snacks. However, make sure these are healthy snacks like fresh pieces of fruits and vegetables. Also avoid creating a pattern of eating lots of different snacks throughout the day. This can develop some bad habits and slow down the weight loss process. Instead, two-three healthy snacks per day will be enough.

Only healthy, solid food should be on your menu. Some basic principles of healthy eating are described at the end of this book.

Another important eating habit you have to adopt is eating slowly and chewing for a long time. Take small bites of solid foods and make sure to chew them 15-20 times before swallowing. This will give your organism more time to digest and you will feel full with less food. The minute you feel full, stop eating! This is a general rule everyone has to adopt, but especially people recovering from the gastric bypass surgery.

When it comes to types of food, make sure always to eat your proteins first. Only after you finish with these, you can move on to vegetables and other carbs. Naturally, your proteins must come from healthy sources like lean meat, poultry, fish, and eggs. All meat cuts on your plate must have their fats removed. This also includes the skin which is extremely fatty and unhealthy. Avoid it!

Drink a lot! Your fluids have to be based on water, unsweetened juices, fat-free broth, and other healthy drinks. However, keep in mind that you must not combine drinks and food. Wait for about 30 minutes to 1 hour after the meal to have your drink.

Make sure to increase your vitamin and mineral intake. You might add some supplements to your daily menu.

Below, you will find some basic healthy recipes to help you get started with your new, healthy life.

Braised Spinach and Leeks

Ingredients:

12 oz fresh spinach, finely chopped

3 large leeks, finely chopped

2 red onions, finely chopped

1 garlic clove, crushed

½ cup cottage cheese

1 tbsp extra virgin olive oil

½ tsp sea salt

Preparation:

Combine spinach and leeks in a large colander. Rinse well under cold running water and drain. Finely chop it and set aside.

Peel the onions and finely chop it. Set aside.

Heat up the olive oil over a medium-high heat. Add sliced leek, garlic, and onions. Stir-fry for about five minutes, over a medium heat.

Now, add spinach and give it a good stir. Season with sea salt and continue to cook for 3 more minutes, stirring constantly.

Remove from the heat and top with cottage cheese

Serve immediately.

Spring Vegetable Soup

Ingredients:

1 medium-sized carrot, finely chopped

2 spring onions, finely chopped

1 yellow bell pepper, finely chopped and seeds removed

2 celery stalks, finely chopped

½ cup celery leaves, finely chopped

½ tsp dried thyme

1 tsp vegetable oil

4 cups vegetable broth

1 cup milk, fat-free

1 tsp salt

Preparation:

Wash and peel the carrot. Finely chop it and set aside. If you are using organic carrot, then don't peel.

Wash the spring onions under cold running water and finely chop it. Set aside.

Wash the bell pepper and cut lengthwise in half. Scoop out the seeds and finely chop it. Set aside.

Wash the celery stalks and finely chop it both, stalks and leaves.

Heat up the oil in a large, heavy-bottomed pan over a medium-high heat. Add finely chopped carrot, spring onions, bell pepper, and celery stalks. Cook for ten minutes, stirring constantly.

Pour in vegetable broth and bring it to a boil. Reduce the heat to medium and add milk, celery leaves, thyme, salt, and pepper. Cover with a lid and cook for 15 minutes, stirring occasionally.

Lean Ground Beef with Wax Beans

Ingredients:

1 lb lean ground beef

1 lb wax beans, cut into bite-sized pieces

1 small onion, finely chopped

1 tbsp of tomato paste

1 cup vegetable broth

1 garlic cloves, crushed

2 tbsp olive oil

2 tbsp fresh parsley, finely chopped

1 tsp salt

¼ cup cheddar cheese

Preparation:

Wash the beans and cut into bite-sized pieces. Set aside.

Grease a large skillet with olive oil and add onions and garlic. Cook until translucent, stirring constantly. Now add ground beef, tomato paste, chopped parsley, and salt. Continue to cook for ten more minutes.

Finally, add wax beans and beef broth. Give it a good stir and cook for 10 more minutes.

Top with cheddar cheese before serving.

Marinated Sea Bream

Ingredients:

2 medium-sized Sea breams, fresh and cleaned

1 cup freshly squeezed lemon juice

1 tbsp fresh rosemary, finely chopped

1 tsp fresh sage, finely chopped

¼ tsp dried thyme, ground

1 tsp sea salt

Preparation:

Wash the fish properly under cold running water. Pat dry with a kitchen paper and set aside.

In a small bowl, combine lemon juice with chopped rosemary, sage, thyme, and salt. Brush the fish with the mixture, especially inside. Stuff each fish with 1-2 rosemary sprigs and secure with toothpicks. Refrigerate for 30 minutes.

Preheat a large, non-stick grill pan or an electric grill. Remove the fish from the refrigerator and grill for 7-10 minutes. Turn once and grill for five more minutes.

Gently remove toothpicks and serve the fish immediately.

Braised Spinach and Leeks

Ingredients:

4 oz kale, chopped

4 oz spinach, chopped

4 oz collard greens, chopped

2 oz Swiss chard, chopped

2 oz parsley leaves, finely chopped

1 medium-sized leek, chopped

1 tbsp olive oil

1 cup vegetable broth

1 tsp sea salt

Preparation:

Wash all greens thoroughly under cold running water and drain in a large colander. Using a sharp knife, chop the vegetables and set aside.

Grease a heavy-bottomed pan with olive oil and add greens. Pour in vegetable broth and season with salt. Bring it to a boil and simmer for 5 minutes.

Serve warm or cold.

Chicken Wings Stew

Ingredients:

2 lbs chicken wings

2 medium-sized potatoes, cut into chunks

2 large fire-roasted tomatoes, chopped

1 large carrot, cut into chunks

2 garlic cloves, finely chopped

2 tbsp of olive oil

1 tsp of smoked paprika, ground

6 cups of chicken broth

2 tbsp of fresh parsley, finely chopped

1 tsp of salt

Preparation:

Rinse the chicken wings under cold running water and pat dry with a kitchen paper. Rub with salt, pepper, and smoked paprika. Set aside.

Peel the potatoes, carrot, and tomatoes. Wash and chop into bite-sized pieces or chunks.

Combine all ingredients in a deep, heavy bottomed pot. Bring it to a boil and reduce the heat to medium-low. Cook for 3 hours.

The recipe tastes even better in a slow cooker. If you own one, cook for 6-8 hours over low heat.

When done, remove the meat from the bones and finely chop. Serve.

Colorful Spring Soup

Ingredients:

1 cup of green peas, pre-cooked

1 large carrot, finely chopped

2 medium-sized red bell pepper, finely chopped

1 cup wax beans, cut into bite-sized pieces

1 medium-sized tomato, roughly chopped

4 cups vegetable broth

1 tbsp olive oil

1 tsp salt

¼ tsp dried oregano, ground

Preparation:

Wash and prepare the vegetables. Peel the carrot and finely chop. With a sharp knife, cut bell pepper in half and remove the seeds. Finely chop. Gently dice the tomato making sure you keep the liquid. Set aside.

Grease the bottom of a deep pan with oil and add chopped carrots, red bell pepper, and wax beans. Stir-fry for five minutes over medium heat. Now add tomato and season with salt and oregano. Continue to cook until all the liquid evaporates.

Finally, pour in vegetable broth and green peas. Bring it to a boil and cook for 10 minutes.

Grilled Chicken Breast

Ingredients:

1 lb chicken breast, sliced into half-inch thick slices

1 cup olive oil

½ cup freshly squeezed lime juice

½ cup parsley leaves, finely chopped

3 garlic cloves, crushed

1 tbsp cayenne pepper

1 tsp dried oregano

1 tsp sea salt

Preparation:

Rinse the meat under cold running water and drain in a large colander. Using a sharp knife, slice into approximately half-inch thick slices. Set aside.

In a medium-sized bowl, combine olive oil with lime juice, chopped parsley, crushed garlic, cayenne pepper, oregano, and salt.

Submerge fillets in this mixture and cover. Refrigerate for 30 minutes.

Preheat a non-stick grill pan over a medium-high heat. Remove the meat from the refrigerator and drain. Grill for 5-7 minutes, turning once.

Mesclun Salad with Mussels

Serves: 4

Preparation time: 10 minutes

Cooking time: 25 minutes

Ingredients:

1 lb fresh mussels, debearded

½ cup onions, peeled and finely chopped

2garlic cloves, crushed

5 tbsp of olive oil

1 tbsp fresh parsley, finely chopped

1 tbsp fresh rosemary, finely chopped

½ cup of lamb's lettuce

½ cup of arugula leaves

1 medium cherry tomato, optional

Salt to taste

Preparation:

Rinse mussels under cold running water. Drain in a large colander and set aside.

In a large, heavy-bottomed pan, heat up 2 tbsp of olive oil over medium-high temperature. Peel and finely chop the onion.

Reduce the heat to medium and add the onions. Stir-fry for several minutes, until crisp-tender. Now add mussels and finely chopped parsley. Cook for 20 minutes, shaking the skillet regularly. When all the water has evaporated, add garlic, chopped rosemary and mix well again.

In a large bowl, combine the mussels with lamb's lettuce. Add the remaining oil, sprinkle with some salt, and decorate with one cherry tomato. Serve immediately.

Cod with Fire-Roasted Tomatoes

Ingredients:

1 cup diced fire roasted tomatoes

2 lbs cod fillet

1 tbsp dried basil

6 cups fish stock

6 tbsp homemade tomato paste

6 chopped celery stalks

3 chopped carrots

½ cup of olive oil

1 finely chopped onion

6 garlic cloves, crushed

½ cup of button mushrooms

Salt and pepper to taste

Preparation:

Wash the fillets thoroughly under cold running water. Pat dry using a kitchen paper and set aside.

Heat up the olive oil in a frying pan, over a medium temperature. Add chopped celery, onions, and carrots. Stir well and cook for about 8-10 minutes. Remove from the heat and transfer to a deep pot.

Add the remaining ingredients and cook for about 15 minutes, over a medium temperature. Stir occasionally.

Serve warm.

Lean Chicken and Vegetable Risotto

Serves: 2

Preparation time: 5 minutes

Cooking time: 25 minutes

Ingredients:

1 cup of rice

½ cup of green beans, pre-cooked

½ cup of sweet corn, pre-cooked

1 medium-sized carrot, sliced

1 medium-sized piece of chicken breast, boneless and skinless

3 tbsp of extra virgin olive oil

½ tsp of salt

Preparation:

Place the rice in a deep pot. Add 2 cups of water and bring it to a boil. Reduce the heat and cook until the water evaporates. Stir occasionally.

Stir in the olive oil, salt, sliced carrot, green beans, and sweet corn. Add one cup of water and continue to cook for another 10 minutes.

Meanwhile, heat up a non-stick frying pan. Place the chicken breast and cover. Cook for 15 minutes, or until the meat has softened. Serve with rice.

Classic Ragout Soup

Ingredients:

1 lb lamb chops (1 inch thick)

1 cup of peas, rinsed

4 medium-sized carrots, peeled and finely chopped

3 small onions, peeled and finely chopped

1 large potato, peeled and finely chopped

1 large tomato, peeled nad roughly chopped

3 tbsp of extra virgin olive oil

1 tbsp of cayenne pepper

1 tsp of salt

½ tsp of freshly ground black pepper

Preparation:

Wash the meat thoroughly under cold running water and pat dry with a kitchen paper. Cut meat into bite-sized pieces and set aside.

Grease the bottom of a deep pot with one tablespoon of olive oil. Make the first layer in the pot with meat. Now add peas, finely chopped carrots, onions, potatoes, and roughly chopped tomato.

Add the remaining olive oil, 2 cups of water, cayenne pepper, salt, and pepper. Give it a good stir and bring it to a boil. Reduce the heat to low and cook for 1 hour.

Remove from the heat and set aside to cool for a while before serving.

Eating Healthy for The Rest of Your Life

Now that your body has fully recovered and changed, it's time to adopt some healthy eating habits for the rest of your life. Remember - your health is defined by the choices you make, so make sure they're healthy ones. Your body goes through millions of processes of digestion and metabolism throughout the day to make you function properly. This is a 24/7 process. If you aren't controlling your diet plant, it's very difficult to see weight loss occurring. But the good news is that if you know what to do on the nutrition front, weight loss is going to feel a hundred times easier than ever before, and you are going to notice:

- you have stable energy levels

- you gain strength faster

- you recover quicker

- you'll be putting your best foot forward at preventing disease development

Nutrition is a game changer for promoting a healthy and fit lifestyle, but most people don't know what it mean to eat properly. You have read a million different diet plans before, but you are still missing the mark on 'healthy' eating. Many of the approaches out there are based more around fad diets and going to extremes just to shed a few pounds, instead of actually promoting weight loss that lasts, and supports optimal health. Thus, there is no escaping the fact that nutrition plays a critical role in your ability to manage your weight. It's time to focus more on eating right for the long-term.

Nutrients in foods that provide the body with calories include:

• Carbohydrates

• Protein

• Fat

When it comes to a healthy diet, the key lies in the balance – eating a range of foods in the right proportions and amounts to maintain a healthy body weight. Food impacts you on critical cellular levels and affects the function of your genes. This, in turn, is one of the key determining factors of aging and poor health. The good news is you can dramatically change your health by adopting a nutrition plan. By following healthy ways of eating, you can maintain health and manage weight. Eating a range of foods reduces your risk of getting certain health conditions, such as heart disease, diabetes, cancer, and osteoporosis. However, by eating a range of foods, I mean healthy foods. There are some foods you should still be avoiding:

- non-toasted bread, especially soft and white

- over-cooked pasta and boiled rice

- red meat with a fibrous texture like steak and chops

- stringy vegetables like green beans

- sweetcorn, pineapple and mushrooms with a toughened texture

- pips, seeds and skins from fruit and vegetables

- dried fruits

But when it comes to healthy eating habits, there are some basic rules you will have to adopt. These simple nutritional tips will help your body digest the food easier and function properly.

1. Drink at least 10, 8oz glasses of water per day Tip 2: Try to nourish your body every 2-4 hours

2. Include a source of protein in every meal

3. Don't skip Breakfast

4. Don't skip lunch, as it will leave you hungrier for dinner with the potential to over eat

5. If you make a mistake, its ok, just be sure to rebound from it and continue the rest of the day with healthy choices

6. No sugary foods or drinks at night

7. Plan a little bit every day, have an idea of what you will eat for all your meals

Once you've adopted these healthy eating habits, you'll find that a healthy eating and maintaining your body weight can be as easy as breathing. A proper diet is really nothing to be afraid of – it is a pure science and an easy one. But to understand things even better, I will go through some basic facts about the macro nutrients your body needs daily. So let's get started...

Macro Nutrients

As I said earlier, you need certain nutrients in the body to get calories (energy). Macronutrients are nutrients needed in large amounts to provide your body with energy to maintain key functions and carry out your daily activities. Carbs, proteins, and fats are 3 essential macronutrients that are responsible for vital functions in the body.

In order for you to understand the basis of correct and healthy eating, you must know the basics of what each of these macronutrients are and what they do. If you do not, you will just fall prey to powerful marketing, which essentially 'banks' on your ability to NOT understand nutrition. Here's what you need to know. . .

Protein

Ideally your diet should comprise at least 30 percent proteins, which are broken down to amino acids in the gut. Your protein intake should be at least 0.8g/kg of bodyweight, though it may vary from person to person, depending on activity levels.

The need for dietary protein are the sought after amino acids. The body uses the amino acids:

- As a light/moderate energy source.

- Building blocks of DNA and muscle tissue

- As building blocks of proteins required by the body for the growth and repair of tissues, boosting immune function, and production of essential enzymes and hormones.

- As the starting material to produce other compounds.

Proteins derived from animal sources have all the essential amino acids required by the body. During digestion, the amount of calories burned by proteins to produce energy is three to four times faster than other macronutrients, including carbohydrates and fat. The more muscle your body has, the greater the amount of calories your body burns on a daily basis. Those who neglect sufficient protein intake, while still being able to lose weight with exercise and a sensible diet, are more likely to experience a higher body fat percentage and lower body weight than those who consume adequate protein amounts for their body and activity levels.

Your best sources of protein are as follows:

• White meat poultry - chicken, turkey

• Seafood - tilapia, salmon, haddock, grouper, mahi, shrimp, etc.

- Lean beef - lean cuts of cow (flank, eye of round, lean ground beef), venison, buffalo. NY strip, porterhouses, skirt, filet mignon, and ribeye's are still acceptable, however, just watch your portion size and weekly consumption. All is needed is 4-6 oz, not the 12-16 oz you get served at restaurants.

- Eggs - both the yolk and the white. Don't worry, it was widely regarded that the yolks caused increased cholesterol, however, that is a myth that has since been disproven by science. The AHA says you can have 1-2 whole eggs per day.

- Pork tenderloin - it is the leanest cut from pork. Stay away from bacon and sausage.

- Legumes - beans

- Soy - tofu

- Dairy - Milk, Cheese, yogurt. While these do contain moderate amounts of protein, they also contain higher amounts of fat per gram or ounce than the rest on this list. Eat these sensibly and in moderation.

Carbohydrates

When creating an optimum nutrition plan for you and your family, you may find it extremely challenging to manage carbohydrate intake. And why? After all, grains have been seen as the base of the outdated food pyramid for decades.

The fact is, our bodies only need a moderate amount of carbohydrates. Of course, the more physically active you are, the higher your requirement for carbohydrates becomes. Generally, your diet should comprise 35-55 percent carbohydrates.

As the main source of energy in the body, carbohydrates are broken down into glucose - the fuel needed by the body to produce energy for the heart, brain, and central nervous system.

You can find carbohydrates in most vegetables, fruits, breads, and grains. Carbohydrates can be found in the majority of foods on the shelves and in our homes. But how do we know what are good and bad carbs? In simple terms, anything that offers calories (even with small amounts) but offer NO nutritional value (ex. Cake, cookies, white bread, soda, chips, 100 calorie snack bags) could be considered 'bad carbs.'

Your carbohydrate sources should be coming from veggies, fruits, and whole grains. It is from non-starchy vegetables that you should get the bulk of your carbohydrate intake. As these vegetables have a relatively modest carbohydrate count compared to grains and starchy veggies, they offer a greater nutrient load than the latter.

While it is pertinent to eat more non- starchy vegetables because they offer fewer calories and more fiber to keep us fuller longer, they also offer a much greater nutrient load from vitamins and minerals. Vitamins, minerals, potassium, antioxidants, and phytonutrients are predominantly found in the vegetables we eat. It is thus important to increase your vegetable consumption to increase your vitamin and mineral concentrations (termed micronutrients) in your body leading to stronger immune support, enhanced blood circulation, stronger bone and joint support, and better cognitive function.

Fat

Dietary fat is different than your body fat. It would seem that the lack of knowledge of nutrition scares most to think dietary fat is bad. It can be considered word and image association where you hear the word "fat" and automatically associate it with the fat on your belly. This is not correct. There are two different types of fats - healthy and unhealthy fats. Healthy fats include seeds, nuts, and unrefined oils and naturally occurring fats in vegetables and meats. The key lies in maintaining moderation and optimizing nutritional benefits. Experts recommend that fats and oil should suffice for at least 10–40 percent of your regular energy needs.

Though fats have earned a poor reputation for their effect on heart health and obesity, some fat is essential for health and wellbeing. Fats help in the absorption of carotenoids and fat-soluble vitamins – A, D, E, K. They supply essential fatty acids needed by the body, which it can't make on its own – like omega-3, an unsaturated fat we must consume. Omega-3 is found in fatty fish meat like salmon.

Fats have the potential to harm as well as help our health. This depends on their fatty acid composition, nutritional value, and their condition. When used in natural, unadulterated state, fat offers optimal nutritional benefits. On the other hand, a very-low-fat diet can compromise our health and ability to lose weight. Monounsaturated and polyunsaturated fats are categorized as "good"; because they help lower cholesterol levels and thus helping reduce the risk for heart disease and diabetes. If your body is deficient in good fats, it can result in obesity, chronic fatigue, and heart problems. Yes, heart ailments from not having enough fat, which have long been associated only with high fat levels. Very important type of polyunsaturated fats, omega-3 fatty acids are especially important for your heart health as they help reduce blood pressure and protect against coronary artery disease. Besides fatty fish, this type of fat can also be found in plant sources like flax seed and chia seeds.

The message I would like you to get is that you don't have to be avoiding fats in order to maintain your hardly won weigh loss – you simply have to choose your fats carefully and eat only what is good for you. It's the only formula for long-term success!

Achieving and Maintaining your Goal Weight

The most important part of your weight loss journey is setting up your goals. If you fail to set a clear goal, it's likely that you will fail to achieve your long-term weight results. Having a firm goal in mind also motivates you to move ahead in your weight loss journey. Consider both – short and long-term goals. Your success depends on setting goals that really matter to you.

Short term goals help you baby-step your way to attainable targets and keep the frustrations low. Clearly defined regular objectives in sight; these goals help you stick to your routine and apprise yourself of daily progress. Creating short-term goals is a smart way of sticking to a daily plan consistently and appropriately, adjusting your diet plan and physical activity into your busy day. When making your short term goals, you must take a note of these additional essentials:

- Eating at a specific time

- Types of food you eat and avoid

- Including a moderate physical activity in your daily schedule

- Writing down your moods and cravings

No matter what your starting point, reaching your short-term goals will make you feel good and give you confidence to progress toward your long-term goals.

After you have succeeded in your short-term goals, it's time to set up long term goals. These goals mean you have a long-term stimulus and target in place and now you need to follow the structured path to reach that goal. Set up your goals clearly and write them down on a paper. This will help you stay motivated and achieve long-term results. As with anything else, the psychology is important. Stay motivated by reminding yourself the benefits. Ensure that your weight loss goals don't create anxiety, stress or pressure. You've been through a lot of stress in the past couple of weeks in order to get the health you deserve! You did a great job and you're finally on the road of a complete life change. This should keep you motivated. Take all the time you need to achieve each one of your goals, you're already half-way there! Remember that!

Including Exercise in Your New Lifestyle

We often hear people advising one another about how to stay fit, be toned, to look slim and adopt wellness as the cardinal principle of life. We also promise to ourselves to adhere to health and fitness regimens the very next day. However, our senses fall prey to temptation of food and the lack of exhaustive workouts. This sets us up, (without control) for bad patterns, ill health and weight gain. The enticement of sleep keeps us bed-bound and we prefer to rest, watch TV and eat a few extra calories with the resolve to start a rigorous workout the next day.

We repeat it every day and fail to tap an embracing working model that supports both our day-to-day goal for fitness and well-being even if we do exercise or engage in vigorous, leisure-time physical activity, we fail to do it frequently. Excuses and fittingly self- justifications keep us away from regular workouts. Weather often becomes a recipe of inactivity and we succumb to the urge to stay inside.

When putting together your workout routine, the first major component you need to figure out is your exercise frequency. The question looks pretty broad when you are forced to think, what type of workouts should be done, and how often will we do any form of exercise: every day, every week and every month? When making these plans you have to keep in mind some important factors that will make your physical activity easy and fun. Keep in mind:

- Your physical condition

- Fitting the exercise into your daily schedule

- Your exercise preferences

- Workout frequency

As someone who's been through a lot lately, your physical condition is probably not at its best. You might want to take things slowly. Any kind of regular physical activity will increase your endurance. It only takes some time so be patient. Remember, even a small house work or an afternoon walk counts as a physical activity. Your body is recovering and soon enough you will be ready for a regular exercise that will keep your body and weight in check.

Some people like smaller exercises every day, others prefer 2-3 times of vigorous exercise per week. Whatever you prefer, make no doubt about one thing – in order to see some exercise results, you need to exercise regularly (on average at least three times a week for optimal progress to be seen and to remain fit. Seniors, who are mostly retired and sedentary, are usually prescribed to at least 30 minutes of jogging or heightened, yet unstressed physical activity every day. Adults, specifically within 18 to 60 years, should embark on 150 minutes of a moderate workout or 75 minutes of vigorous physical activity each week. Healthcare experts have agreed in their suggestion that it should be spread over at least three days each week and for 10 to 20 minutes each activity at one go. However, you stand to gain more health benefits when active five hours each week. To add to it, you should also focus strengthening activities for a minimum of twice a week. According to a recent study published in the journal; Applied Physiology, Nutrition and Metabolism, "adults should aim to accumulate at least 150 minutes of weekly physical activity in whatever pattern that works for their schedule."

Now the main question here is what type of workouts should you do in order to maintain the weight you hardly won. The answer is simple. You engage in a number of physical activities in your day-to-day life. Have you ever imagined how many calories you burn while climbing stairs or gardening? These small, but useful steps are in the right direction.

The more you move your body, the more fat you burn. Continuing this more frequently in your everyday life offers advantages. Strength and stretching exercises at leisure help keep muscles strong and flexible. Jogging, swimming and biking are called aerobic exercises, which are essential to keep your heart healthy and improve stamina. The more frequent these are, the better placed your health and wellness.

The time available for workout has two aspects. First, you always seem to be in a hurry thanks to the piling household chores, burdens at work, family, and the way we are used to living "the busy life." Second, whenever the time is available, we are more amenable to planning for the next day or making excuses than doing the workout.

If you are serious, start now and forget excuses. If unable to do so, you still have a way to get rid of both the time factor and procrastination.

The following are 12 easy ways to make time for regular exercise and beat the time crunch:

1. Never wait for big amounts of time to break the ground. Start immediately and in short bursts.

2. Create 10-minute segments every morning and evening prior to your meal for an intense aerobic workout.

3. Utilize every possible opportunity to walk, ascend stairs and involve in physical activity.

4. Take your child or pet for a brisk walk.

5. Walk and talk. Make it a habit.

6. Think about the fallout of being a couch potato.

7. Spice up your routine by exploring new neighborhoods or turning your walk into a 'scavenger hunt' of your town or city.

8. Walk today, swim tomorrow and go to the gym the day after.

9. If you have a treadmill at home, go for a jog during your TV time.

10. Participate in team sports with family members during holidays.

11. Park your car at a distance and walk to your destination.

12. Shun the elevator and take the stairs.

Ditching the excuses can be the first step to a healthier you. But your workout must be compatible with your physical condition and age. The Human body "rests" as we grow older and loses flexibility. The stamina to bear rigorous exercise also stems down.

Don't compare yourself with others. Set your personal goals for health and fitness, and identify high to moderate or low-impact exercises that you are able to do and willing to enjoy.

Talk to yourself and doctor and make a list of things that work out for you. Make those physical activities routine and take pleasure in them. Of course, as someone who has recently had a serious operation, talk to your doctor first to see if there is a low-impact exercise you can do or find out if you should wait until you are healed.

Just like with nutrition, setting up goals for exercise can have some major benefits. Smartly planed exercise goals will motivate you and keep frustrations low – everything you need for a normal workout consistency. When making your short term goals, you must take a note of these additional essentials:

1. Workout at a specific time

2. Workout for a specific duration

3. What is the exercise for the day (running, weights, cycling, etc.)

4. How much weight to use

5. Number of sets and reps per exercise

6. Rest periods between sets of exercise

7. Nutritional adherence

Choosing the Right Type of Training

Aerobic training, in simple terms, requires you to enhance oxygen consumption at a higher than normal rate. Most common examples are jogging, running, swimming, aerobics, dance, treadmill, climbing up stairs and intense sports.

The meaning of the word aerobic is "living in air." Those exercises that demand higher use of oxygen for metabolism than normal or "lighter activities" are grouped as aerobic training. When you undertake physical activities that go beyond the normal level and involve speed and increasingly intense movements, you begin to breathe more rapidly. The reason is sudden increase in metabolism and fat burning requiring your lungs to supply oxygen at a higher amount, and quickly! Aerobic activities result in an improved heartbeat and flow of blood inside your body. You must have at least three times-a-week intense aerobic activity, at 15-20 minutes per workout to reduce fat, improve mood, make the heart and lungs stronger and cut down the risk of diabetes. Other important benefits include:

- Strengthening of the muscles

- Enhancing metabolism to burn more calories

- Superior respiratory ability

- Improving efficiency and stroke volume of the heart

- Facilitating the flow of air in and out of the lungs

- Increase in red blood cells and oxygen circulation

- Reduced stress and lowering of depression

- Improved cognitive capacity

- Reduced diabetes risk

- Stimulate bone growth

- Enhanced energy molecule storage leading to improved muscle mass

- Greater endurance and mobility

- Improved use of fat and intramuscular glycogen

- Better quality of life

When combined with a moderate anaerobic exercise like weight lifting, you get a valuable exercise plan to keep your health and strengthen your body. Remember, only a proper diet and a regular exercise can give you the results you want!

The last factor that you want to make sure you have in place, and another one that can quickly make or break your program. Fun!

You would be amazed at how many people (and you may be one of them yourself!) that put themselves on a diet and workout program they hate. They force themselves into the gym each and every day, but sooner or later, they just cannot take it anymore. If they have to face one more long-drawn-out session on the treadmill or another go- around with the same weight machine circuit they've been doing for as long as they can remember, they might just scream. This is wrong!

Your workouts must be fun. If you hope to stick with them for longer than a few weeks, enjoying them is critically important.

And while what one person defines as fun may not necessarily be the same as what another person classifies as fun, there are some general principles that will apply to almost everyone.

- Workouts should be:

- Fast paced

- Ever-changing

- Full of new and exciting exercises

- Done in a supportive and energetic environment

If you can satisfy all of these requirements, chances are you will be having yourself a pretty good time while you do your workout. If you're having a good time, you'll also be more likely to make a positive association with exercise in your mind. This is very important as it will encourage you to keep going with those workouts over the long haul. The minute your workout becomes more of a chore – something you dread doing – is the minute that you won't be making fitness a part of your lifestyle for years to come.

If you want to reach your body weight, health, and fitness goals, this needs to be a choice to change your life for the better. You need to want to work out regularly and eat healthy because you like doing so – you feel good when you do it, and you feel even better when you are seeing the results.

Conclusion

Your journey is finally over and you're ready to live a happy and healthy life you deserve. By now have seen what a balanced diet and a proper meal should look like, I hope that it has helped you to realise that a healthy lifestyle is not a magic, but rather a pure science, and a very important science in everyone's life.

Eat more fresh, organic food and avoid those processed, unhealthy meals – as simple as that!

At this point you have seen what some simple, classic ingredients can do when combined together. I hope it made you understand that never again you have to eat unhealthy foods to satisfy your taste. I hope this simple guide brought some improvements into your life – your everyday menu and your entire eating habits. It was created to be a guide in your gastric bypass surgery journey and help you become motivated for the rest of your life.

Read my recipes and implement some of the advice, and stay happy and healthy as you are now!

Make sure to try all of my recipes and leave some comments. Your feedback and comments mean the world to me. Please take a moment and tell me what you think about these meals and preparation methods. Both, positive and negative feedback will challenge me to write more efficiently in the future.

Thank you for taking the time to go through this book and enjoy your new and healthy lifestyle!

Wish you all the best,

Luke Newman

Check out this book!

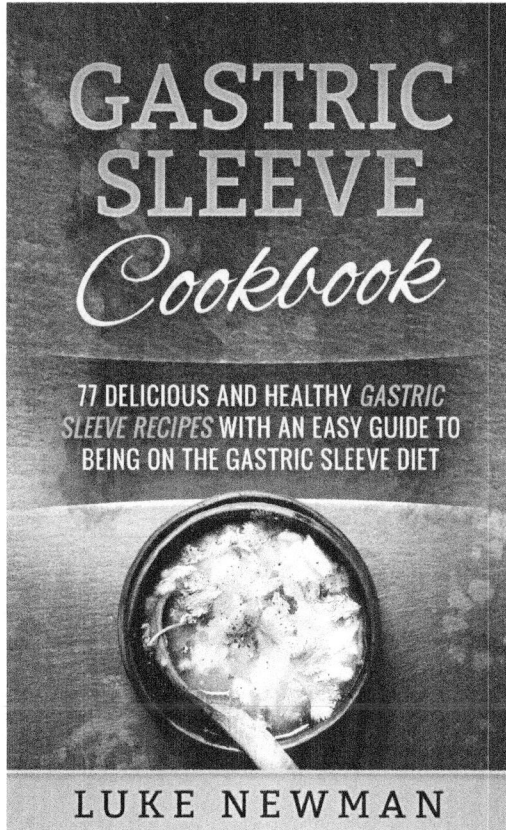

GASTRIC SLEEVE *Cookbook*

77 DELICIOUS AND HEALTHY *GASTRIC SLEEVE RECIPES* WITH AN EASY GUIDE TO BEING ON THE GASTRIC SLEEVE DIET

LUKE NEWMAN

Printed in Great Britain
by Amazon

40736311R00096